Clothes Around the World

by Elizabeth Moore

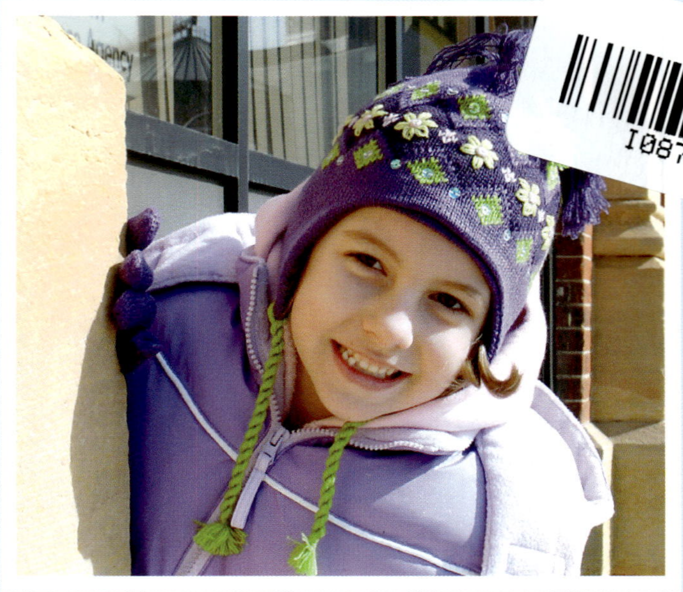

Consultant:
Adria F. Klein, Ph.D.
California State University, San Bernardino

capstone classroom
Heinemann Raintree • Red Brick Learning
division of Capstone

People wear different kinds of clothes.

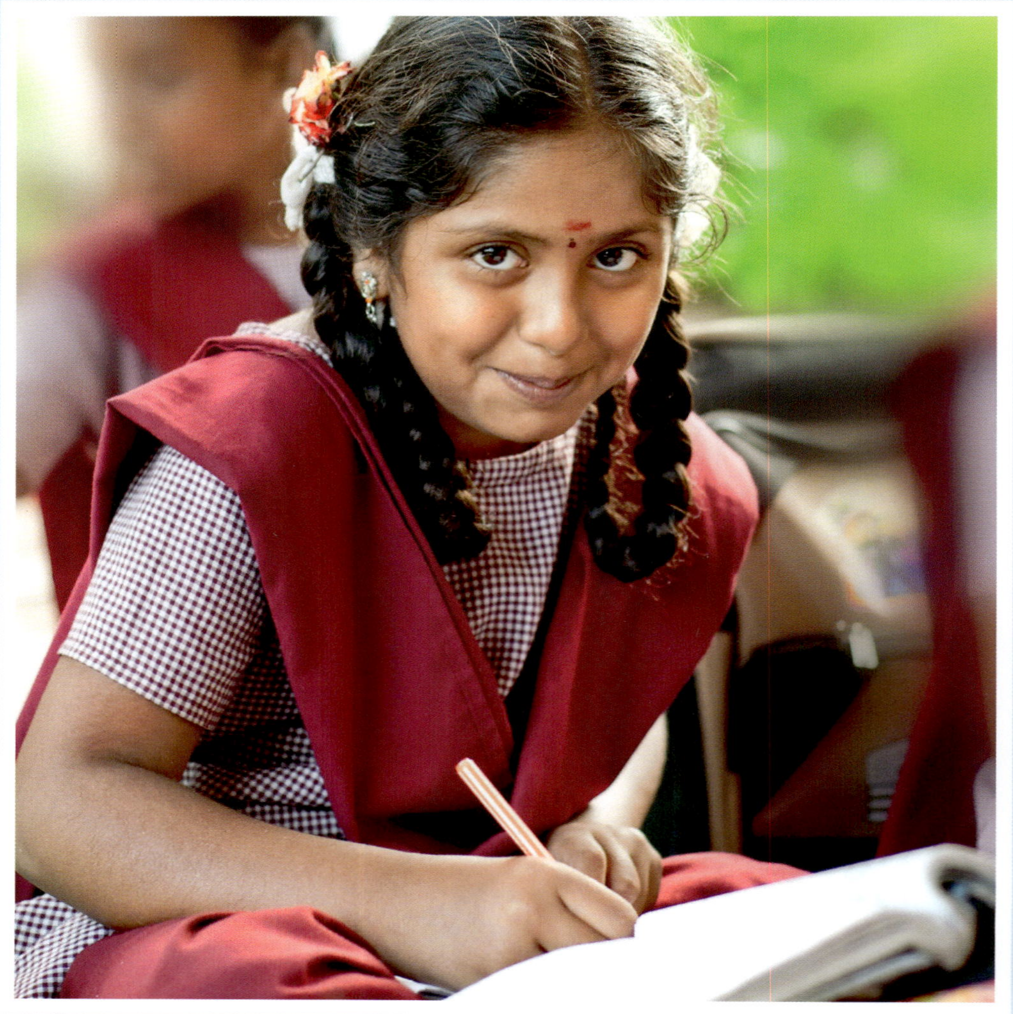

Clothes protect people from cold and heat.

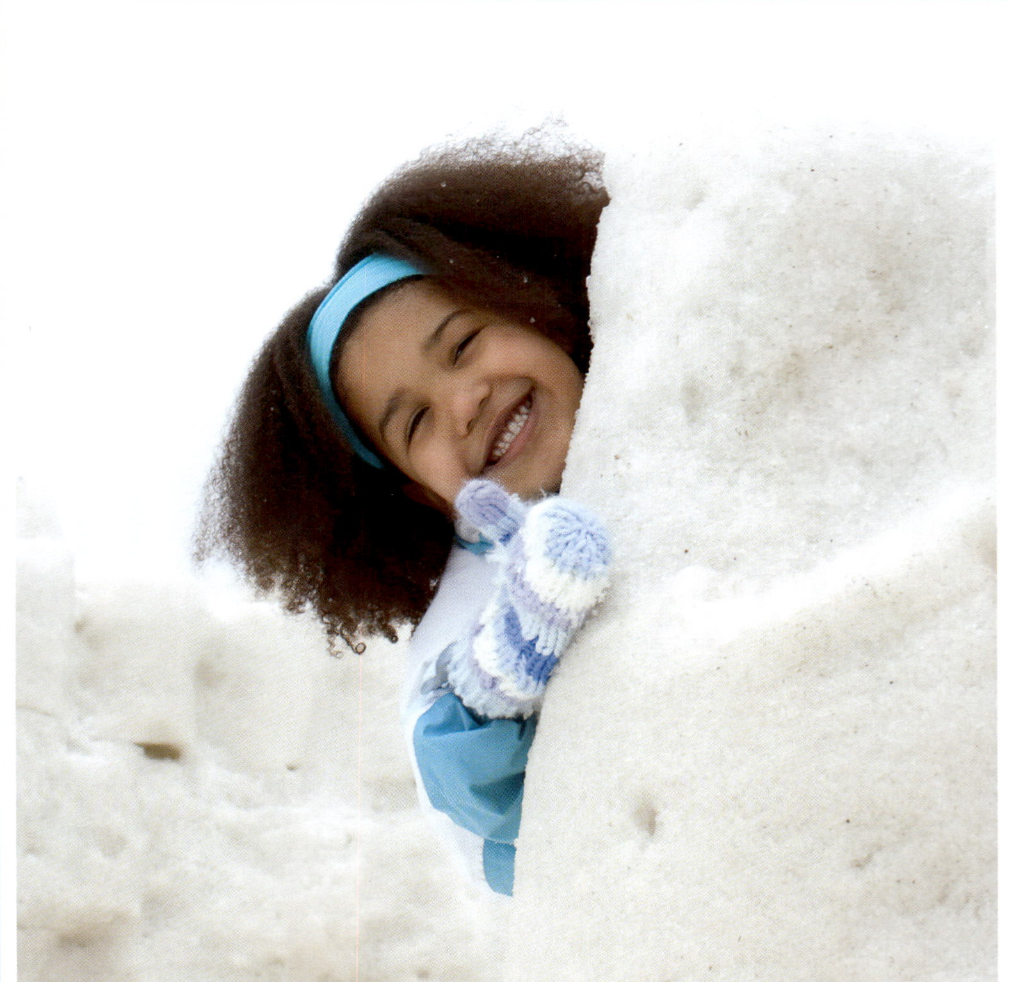

People choose clothes that fit them.

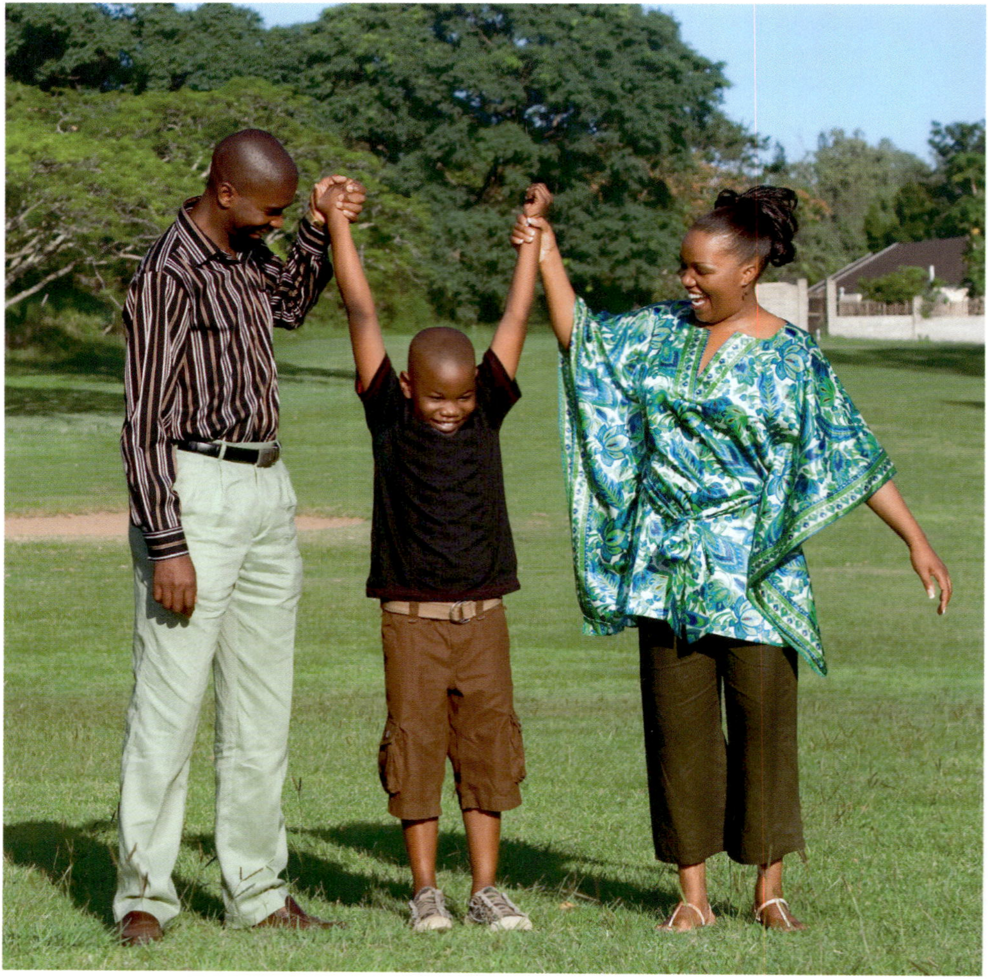

People choose clothes that are best for the weather.

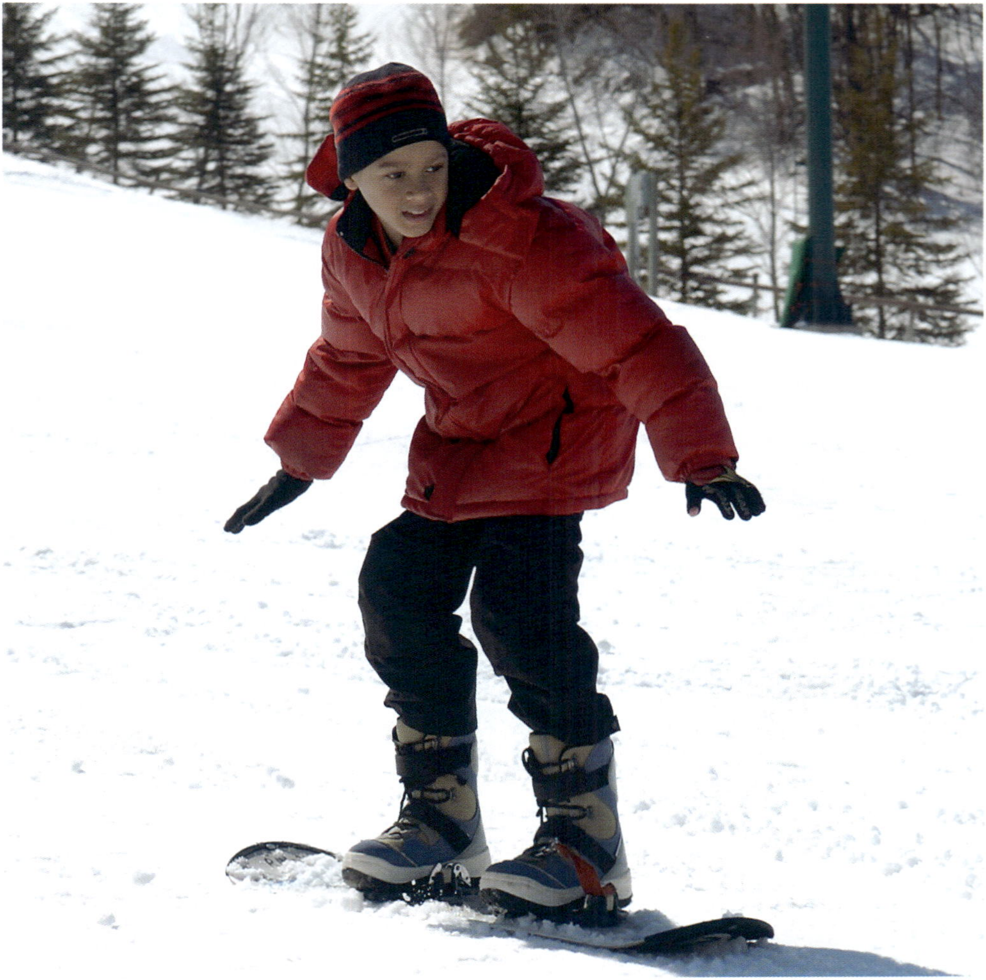

Some places are very hot almost all the time.

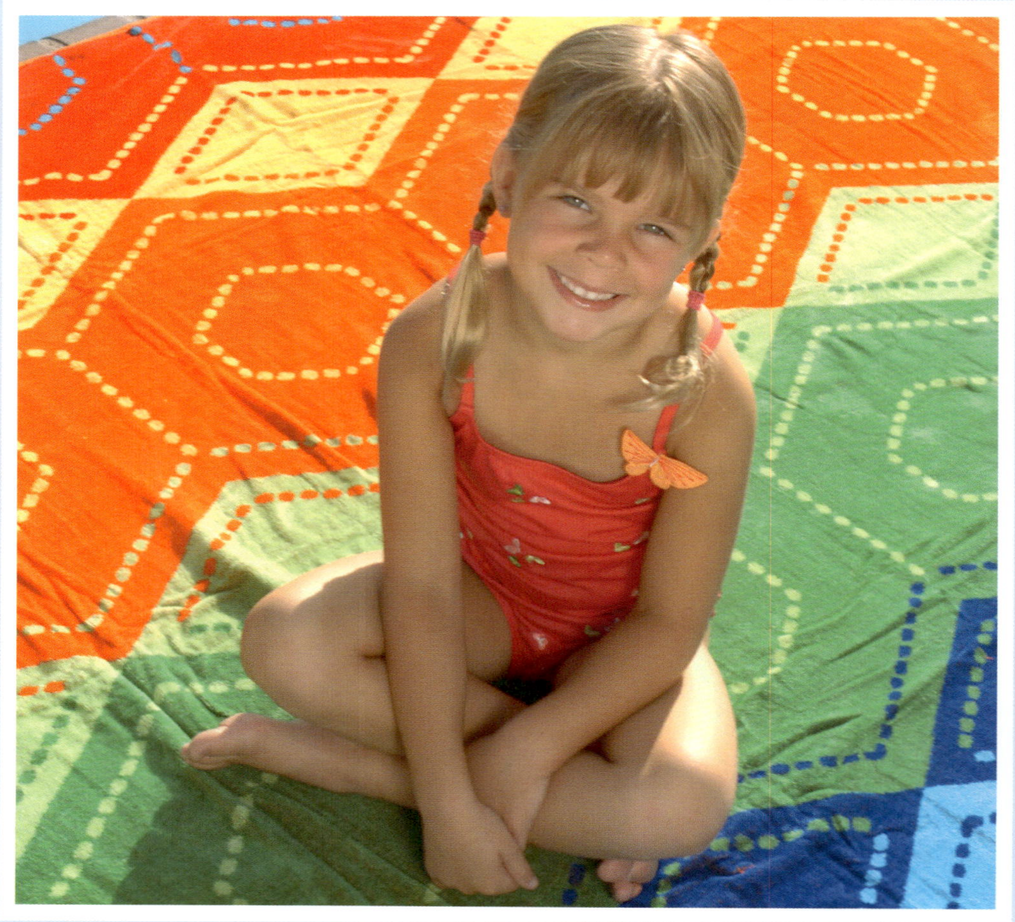

The clothes people wear in hot places protect them from the sun.

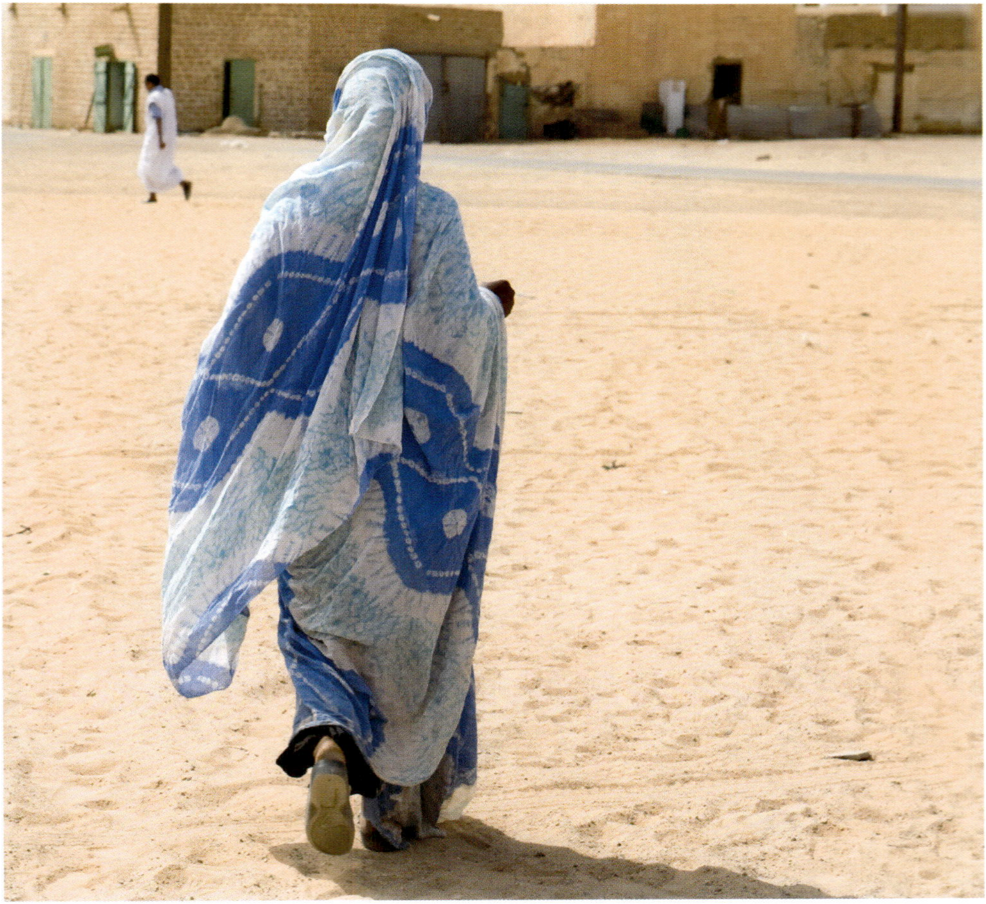

Light colored clothes help people stay cool.

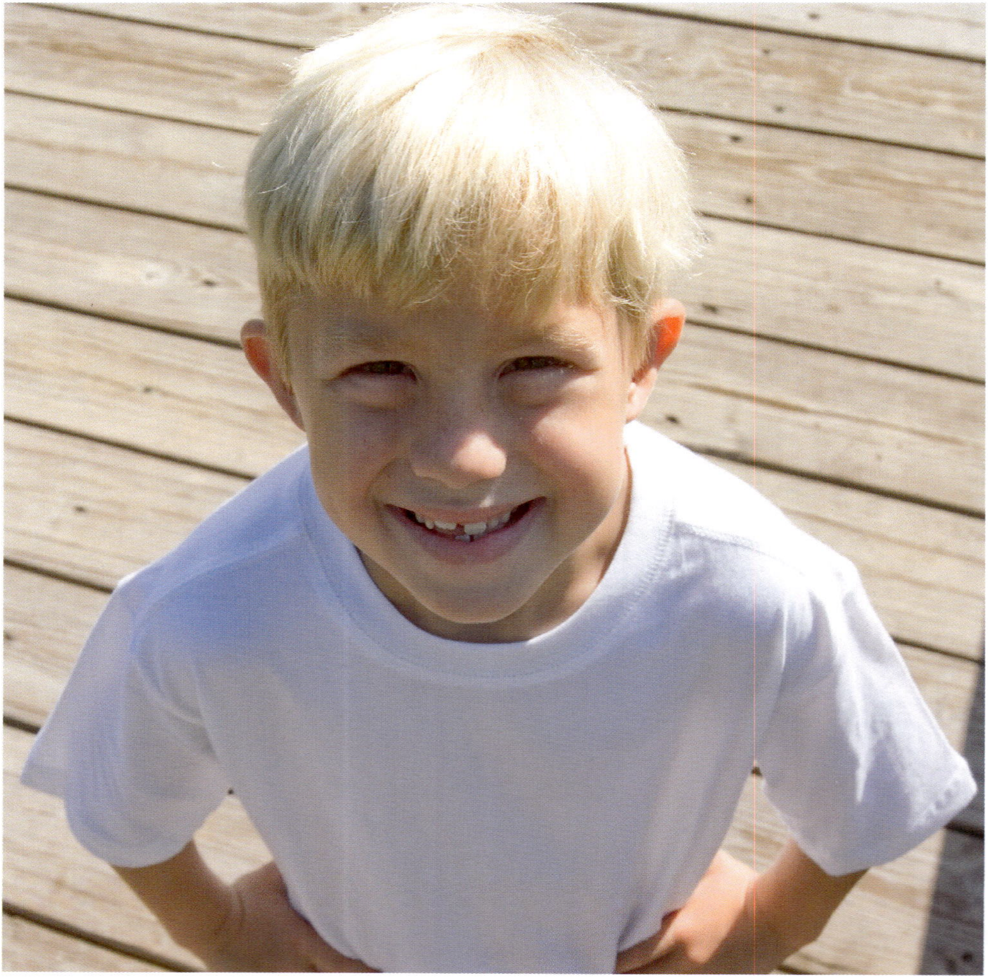